OUTSIDE THE BOX

OUTSIDE THE BOX
A TACTICAL APPROACH TO DEMENTIA CARE

KEVIN WALTERS, LNA

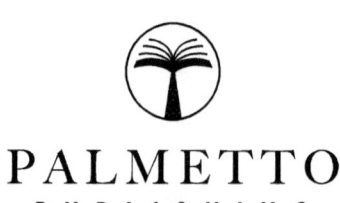

PALMETTO
PUBLISHING
Charleston, SC
www.PalmettoPublishing.com

Copyright © 2024 by Kevin Walters, LNA

All rights reserved.

No portion of this book may be reproduced, stored in a retrieval system, or transmitted in any form by any means–electronic, mechanical, photocopy, recording, or other–except for brief quotations in printed reviews, without prior permission of the author.

Paperback ISBN: 979-8-8229-4857-0
eBook ISBN: 979-8-8229-4858-7

Cover Photo by ImaJenAtion.com

This book is dedicated to all of my co-workers who unselfishly put their best foot forward in providing care to residents living with dementia; this includes all shifts and all positions. Without their teamwork, their patience, and their unselfish dedication to duty, every day would be just another long, nameless day for the residents.

There are far too many people to thank, but I will send a shout out to Deloris, the lead nurse on my unit who inspired the book's title. On every review she gave me, she commented on how I like to "...think outside the box...". Again, thank you to everyone.

A special thanks also goes out to all the residents' family members and friends who took time out of their busy schedules to visit their loved ones. They brought so much love and compassion with each and every visit. They understood and appreciated the tactical approaches we used in caring for their loved ones; many of them adopted a tactical approach of their own. I overheard one visitor say something to his loved one just as he was leaving: "I have to go to work now, but I'll be home later." He didn't say he'd be "back" later, he said he'd be "home" later. I can only imagine how reassuring that was to that resident.

Lastly, a special thanks to my own family, who pushed me through to the finish line in writing this book.

TABLE OF CONTENTS

Preface · vii
In the Beginning · 1
Direct versus Tactical · 6
Morning Care · 15
Nutrition · 21
Bathing · 27
Toileting · 30
Medication · 37
Behaviors · 40
Exit Seeking · 42
Wandering and Rummaging · · · · · · · · · · · · · · · · · · 46
Aggression · 49
Repetitiveness · 52
The List Goes On · 56
Building and Maintaining Relationships · · · · · · · · · · · · 57
Summary · 61

PREFACE

In 1987, Congress passed the Nursing Home Reform Act into law. This was done to improve the quality of care and the quality of life offered to residents in nursing homes at the time. The law carried with it a sort of "Resident Bill of Rights."

Most of the rights listed are obvious: the right to clean air and water; the right to privacy; and the right to be free from neglect and abuse. Other rights are a bit more involved, such as the right to self-administer certain medications and the right to be informed of medical conditions. This book was inspired by one particular right that can test the will of any caregiver, myself included: the right to refuse care. According to the bill of rights, any resident has the right to refuse care at any time for any reason.

KEVIN WALTERS, LNA

The incidents and outcomes described in this book are based on my own real-life experiences throughout my career as a licensed nursing aide (LNA). All names have been changed to protect privacy.

The tactics and methods described in this book are *not* intended to diagnose, treat, cure, or prevent dementia in any way. They *are* intended, however, to inspire a new, tactical approach to providing care to residents living with dementia.

IN THE BEGINNING

I began my career as an LNA in 2006 on a long-term care unit. The residents on the unit were there for a number of different reasons—some were there due to terminal illness, cancer, or other chronic conditions that could be better treated at a facility; some were there for physical ailments such as amputated limbs; some were there because of the lack of assistance available from family and friends. Despite their different reasons for being there, though, the residents on the unit all had one thing in common: they all had their wits about them.

Those residents knew they were in a nursing facility and were accepting of the fact that they needed assistance in certain aspects of their daily living. Mary knew she was physically incapable of transferring from her bed to her wheelchair without assistance, and she knew to ring her call-bell for help. Ron knew he needed assistance getting dressed and making his bed, as he had lost one of his hands in a boating accident. Edith knew she had a urinary catheter and that it needed to be checked regularly by the nurse on duty.

Along with knowing the assistance they needed throughout the day and how to ask for it, there was something else they were all aware of—they knew they could refuse care at any time. Posted throughout the facility in big, bold letters on bright yellow paper were three words: NO MEANS NO—you couldn't miss it. Just below those words was an excerpt from the bill of rights regarding a resident's right to refuse care.

Different residents on the unit would refuse different things on different days for different reasons. John might not be very hungry and refuse breakfast; he could always ask a staff member to call the kitchen for a sandwich later in the morning. Janet would often tell the LNAs on duty that she would rather wait until after breakfast to change out of her pajamas. Whatever their reason might be, I was told by my supervisor to respect the residents' rights, simply report any refusals to the charge nurse, and include it in my charting.

After only three months of working on the long-term care unit, just as I was getting a daily rhythm going, I got transferred to the locked-down dementia unit. Once inside the unit, the only way out was with the well-protected combination, known only by employees of the facility and local emergency officials.

I had heard stories about the difficulties that can arise when trying to provide care for the residents on that unit.

There were stories about residents disrobing in public, using trashcans as toilets, and lashing out at staff members. I knew, however, that the more a story gets told over time, the more exaggerated it can get. I was about to find out for myself just how exaggerated the stories had become…or had they?

Just like the residents on the long-term care unit, the residents on this unit all had something in common—they all suffered from some type of dementia. Whether it be Alzheimer's disease, vascular dementia, Lewy body dementia, Parkinson's disease, or any other condition that falls under the dementia umbrella, the mental capacity of every resident on the unit was under attack on a daily basis. Slowly but surely, their learning ability, communication skills, judgment, reasoning, short-term memory, and long-term memory were being wiped away. Also like the long-term care unit, different residents would refuse different things on different days for different reasons.

Unlike refusals I would get on the long-term care unit—which usually came with a reasonable explanation—refusals on this unit were often irrational. Randy refused to get out of his wet pajamas. "They're not wet; they're warm!" he argued. Linda refused to eat her lunch. "I'm not hungry; I'm still full from breakfast," even though she had refused that too. Dennis refused to take his scheduled pain medication when the nurse brought it to him because he wasn't having pain at that very moment. "The pain's already gone; I don't need medicine," he told the nurse.

Again, I was told to report any refusals to the charge nurse and to include it in my charting. I used a lot of ink checking off the box marked, "Resident Refused."

So, how do you get Randy out of his wet pajamas and into some fresh, clean clothes? How do you get 105-pound Linda to eat a healthy meal? How does the unit nurse get Dennis (who suffers from chronic pain) to stop refusing his scheduled pain medicine?

You could try explaining to Randy that his pajamas are wet with urine and that it could cause his skin to break down. Sadly, though, his dementia has minimized his ability to rationalize the situation—the only thing he's concerned with at the moment is how warm his pajamas feel.

You could try reasoning with Linda about the importance of maintaining a healthy weight, but her ability to reason has been compromised by her dementia.

The nurse could inform Dennis that taking his medicine helps to control his pain, but due to his dementia, Dennis is focused only on that very moment—why fix what's not broken?

Professionally, I knew it was my duty to respect the residents' right to refuse; it's written in the law. At the same time, though, I also had an ethical duty to provide the care these residents needed.

Rather than try to explain, reason, inform, or instruct, I decided to adopt a more tactical approach to providing care for these residents; I decided to step outside the box. My philosophy was this: the less I offered my assistance, the less opportunities they would have to refuse. That's not to say I neglected the care they so desperately needed—I simply approached their needs from a different, more tactical angle.

DIRECT VERSUS TACTICAL

Some readers will see the word "tactical" and associate it with words like devious, tricky, deceitful, and dishonest. I would argue that it fits more along the lines of strategic, observant, attentive, or even compassionate.

Understanding there might be less optimistic views of my tactical method, I decided to do a small, unofficial survey among family members who would come to visit their loved ones. I made sure—through my supervisor at the time—that my questions were nonspecific enough to avoid any violations regarding health information and privacy.

I won't go over the specifics of my survey, but I will say an overwhelming majority of those I spoke with agreed with and supported my tactical approach. In fact, one lady, who initially considered my approach "less than honest," changed her view one day while she was visiting with her uncle Joe.

OUTSIDE THE BOX

She approached me in the hallway and told me that her uncle's roommate, Phil, was rummaging through Joe's closet and thought Phil might end up stealing one of her uncle's shirts or something. I explained to her that Phil had recently moved from a room where his closet was to the right of the sink, which is where Joe's closet was—and had been since he moved into the facility. I assured her that Phil's actions were harmless and that all residents' personal belongings were labeled with their name; anything Phil might take out of Joe's closet would be returned to Joe.

This wasn't the first episode of Phil going through Joe's closet or drawers, or even lying on Joe's bed. In the past, other staff and I had tried a more direct approach, saying things like, "Phil, this isn't your bed..."; "Phil, your closet is on the other side..."; or "Mr. Clark, let's leave Mr. Moffett's things alone..." This would usually lead to Phil taking on a defensive stance. Although we were eventually able to coax Phil away from Joe's closet, it often left him feeling degraded or even angry. In his view, we were telling him he was doing something wrong.

This time, though, rather than approaching Phil in a direct manner and risk putting him in a state of distress—or anger—I decided to try a more tactical approach.

Joe's niece and I walked into the room and sure enough, Phil was sifting through Joe's closet. I walked over and started sifting alongside him. "Oh, my goodness,

Phil," I sighed, "did they put your sweater in the wrong closet again? That's the second time this week."

"I can't find it anywhere," Phil answered, still sifting.

"I bet I know what happened..." I sighed again. "...I bet the laundry person forgot you moved to the other side of the room so you could be closer to the door." I walked over to the other closet, opened the door, and grabbed the first sweater I found. I looked at the label and read it out loud. "Phil Clark! Would you look at that!" I pulled the sweater off the hanger and helped him put it on. "Hey, look! They even replaced your missing button."

"Well, that was nice of them," he replied.

"One other thing, Phil," I continued, "I found your missing slippers and wanted to be sure they spelled your name right." I reached into his closet and grabbed his slippers. "Did they spell your last name right?" I asked, handing him the slippers.

"C-L-A-R-K," he spelled out loud. "That's me, alright." He put the slippers on the bottom shelf and closed the closet door. Having him be the one to put the slippers away and close the door was a small first step toward Phil recognizing his own closet. That whole scene took less than five minutes, and everyone was happy. I invited Phil to the dining room for some juice, he accepted, and we were on our way.

By me joining in on the sifting rather than asking him to stop, Phil felt my genuine concern for his situation—the sighing only emphasized my concern. I'm not sure what Phil was actually looking for, but the reference to a sweater gave the search some meaning. The "...wrong closet again..." remark hinted to Phil that this had happened before and that it wasn't his fault. Reading his name out loud and helping him put the sweater on reassured the idea that it actually *was* a sweater he was looking for. The mention of the replaced button—which was never really missing—solidified the sweater theory and even brought a bit of a smile. Mentioning that I was thirsty and inviting Phil to join me moved Phil's focus off of the whole closet incident and onto quenching our thirst. Joe's niece was now a firm believer in the tactical approach.

I could have used the same direct approach with Phil that I had used in the past; I could have been straightforward and factual. I knew from experience, though, how that could affect his mood long into the day.

When someone with dementia gets angry or upset, it can last for hours. It's not because they're holding a grudge—it's because they know they're upset, but they can't remember why. This can leave them feeling even more upset, which can lead to isolation, which can lead to refusing help with personal care, which can then lead to a variety of other health issues.

I feel that most refusals from residents with dementia are fueled by the fact that they don't know—and don't trust—the person offering to assist them. They're in no hurry to let some stranger tell them what they need help with, let alone have that stranger be the one to help them.

For this reason, I cannot stress enough the importance of building and maintaining a relationship with each resident. A friendly relationship not only gives them a sense of belonging, but it can work wonders when it comes to providing care. The importance of relationship can be summed up like this: with relationship comes trust; with trust comes cooperation; with cooperation comes quality care; with quality care comes quality of life…our main goal.

Building these relationships takes some creativity and may require a bit of what I call ethical deception. To give an example, this is how I built a relationship with Jack when he first came to live in the facility. I pulled one of his family members aside and asked where Jack went to school, and they informed me that he was a graduate of Dover High School.

While I was helping to put some of Jack's belongings into his closet, I paused and looked at him with a curious squint. "Jack? Jack Roberts?" I asked. "I thought you looked familiar." I had his attention. "Did you go to Dover High?"

"Yeah, who are you?" he replied, trying to place my face into his memory.

"My name's Kevin," I replied. "We never hung out, but I think you were in my English class." He looked at me again.

"Oh yeah!" he replied. Suddenly he felt less like a stranger, even though we had never gone to school together. The thirty-year age gap between us was irrelevant to Jack; his mind was too busy trying to place me.

Is there a bit of trickery involved with being tactical? Yes. But it is far outweighed by the results. Was I lying when I told Jack we might have been in the same class at Dover High? Yes again. But the gap between us was suddenly made much smaller—I was no longer a stranger.

If you still question the ethical morality of using a tactical approach as opposed to being up front and honest with dementia residents, consider the following true story.

Mary, a widow of many years, who had been on the dementia unit for several months, would often ask me or any other staff member if her husband was around. Sparing her feelings, I would always reply by telling her I hadn't seen him but that I would keep an eye out. If she asked me again a little later, I would give her the same answer. Immediately after every answer, I would sidetrack into a whole different subject. "Is that a new shirt, Mary?" A small one-on-one would ensue and the whole husband search would be ended...for the moment, at least.

One day, just after breakfast, Mary walked up and asked the nurse—who was new to the dementia unit—if her husband was around. Knowing Mary was a widow, the nurse gave her a direct and truthful answer. "I'm sorry, Mary," she said in a gentle, caring voice, "your husband died." Mary walked back to her room, sobbing and sniffling the whole way. In her dementia-riddled mind, she took the nurse's statement as if her husband had died that very day—she was reliving the whole incident of her husband's death all over again. Was the nurse trying to hurt Mary? No, but she thought lying to her was inappropriate.

I could have tried explaining to Mary that her husband had died several years back, but that would only keep her mind on the fact that her husband had died. This situation called for some tactical intervention.

I knocked on Mary's door, entered her room, and closed the curtains. I sat on the chair beside her bed and said to her in a mournful voice, "These rainy days make me a little sad, too, Mary." I grabbed each of us a tissue and continued, "I don't get it," I said to her. "The weather man said it was supposed to be a beautiful, sunny day." I continued my small talk as I walked toward the window. I opened the curtains wide and voila: "Oh my goodness, Mary, the weatherman was right. You have to come see this." She walked to the window to have a look.

"Well, it's about time those weather people get it right." She finished wiping her eyes and handed me her tissue. Her sadness was now due to another rainy day, which was now replaced by a bright, sunny day.

I must confess, the sun had been shining all morning—there wasn't a cloud in the sky. My opening of the curtains, however, combined with my excitement made it as though it was all brand new to both of us.

Without Mary's trust that I earned through the relationship I had built with her, I don't think she would have accepted my compassion so openly; she might have told me to just leave her alone.

I had learned through a coworker that Mary once worked as a middle school teacher. One morning, as I was making her bed, I said to her, "Well, Mary, I got my history test back, and I didn't do so well. I guess I should have studied more, huh?"

"Yes, you should have," she sneered back.

"I can never remember which president freed the slaves," I told her. "Was it Jefferson or Lincoln?"

"It was Abraham Lincoln," she said confidently.

Although I was being "less than honest" about not knowing about Abraham Lincoln and despite the fact that I hadn't taken a history test in over thirty years, the triggering of Mary's intact long-term memory gave her a sense of self-worth; she was helping me with something I couldn't figure out by myself.

With the okay from her family and my supervisor, I added a strip of paper with the words "REST IN PEACE" to the bottom of her late husband's picture. I felt that Mary's dementia might prevent her from comprehending the traditional RIP; she might start wondering, "Who is Rip?" Within just a few days of saying a short prayer with her for her late husband during morning care, Mary's questioning of her husband's whereabouts was put to rest—pun intended.

So, getting back to the subject, what are some things residents might refuse, and how do we avoid those potential refusals? Theoretically, as I mentioned earlier, they can't refuse what we don't offer—that's not to say we ignore their needs; we simply redirect our approach. Instead of offering, we initiate, we encourage, and we stimulate. We use subliminal body language and gestures to invite them to join us in whatever task we are trying to accomplish. Dementia causes their mind to try to focus on one subject at a time. With just a few words, we can steer their attention toward something pleasant—we can direct their mind to a beautiful, sunny day, for instance. It's important to remember, though, it's not us against them, but it's us and them against their dementia. Let's go over some tactics I use throughout a typical day.

MORNING CARE

I'll start with Randy and his "warm" pajamas. My relationship with Randy was built through exchanges about roofing, something we actually had in common. I would ask him questions on certain aspects of roof repair, and he would offer me his expert advice. On occasion I would tell him his advice worked and my roof didn't leak anymore. My roof never leaked in the first place, but you could tell his spirits were lifted—his expert advice had made a difference.

I was told in morning report that the previous shift had attempted to get Randy washed and dressed, but he was not having any part of it. Respecting his right to refuse while also avoiding an angry reaction, they turned off his light and let him be. They were not neglecting his care—they were respecting his rights.

I knocked on the door as I entered the room and turned on the light over Randy's bed. "Sorry I'm late, bud," I said in an out-of-breath manner as I opened his closet and started picking out clothes. "I accidently set my alarm for p.m. instead of a.m."

"Don't worry about it," he replied with a big yawn. "I did the same thing yesterday."

I never mentioned the task at hand; I never told Randy it was time to get out of bed or even that the bed was wet. I entered with a heartfelt apologetic tone and he responded with a "don't worry about it" attitude. I also never mentioned it was time to get dressed. I simply opened his closet and began pulling out clothes, and that action in itself was like a subliminal hint that he picked up right through the alarm clock conversation.

"You'll probably want some warm socks today," I continued, as I turned on the water to fill Randy's wash basin, still sounding out of breath. "Someone said it might be a little chilly today." I put lotion on his feet and put his socks and slippers on. "Does that feel better?"

"Much better," he answered, as he sat up on the side of his bed. Mentioning the warm socks and chilly weather kept Randy's mind occupied with the weather while elusively reinforcing the idea that it was time to get dressed. Also, I find that by asking if something feels "better" (like I did with the slippers) as opposed to feeling "good," residents tend to respond more positively. I have no explanation as to why—perhaps the word good is too subjective, or maybe the word better implies an improvement. Randy said the slippers felt better even though there was nothing to compare them to.

"Let me make sure nobody's in the bathroom." I knocked on the door, waited a couple of seconds, and then slowly opened the bathroom door to peek inside. "It's all yours." I knew ahead of time that there was nobody in the bathroom; however, the curiosity caused by me knocking on the door, followed by confirming that it was "all his," prompted Randy into the bathroom.

"The laundry girl should be here any minute now," I told him. "We better put these pajamas in your laundry basket before she gets here." I put his wet pajamas in a plastic bag and placed a towel over his lap, asking him to hold it there for me. I told him I would let him sit and do his business in private. I stepped out of the bathroom, leaving the door cracked just enough where I could stay out of Randy's line of sight while still being able to see if he was staying seated. He felt his privacy, and I felt close enough to intervene if needed.

We got washed and dressed and headed for the dining room. "We better get to the dining room while breakfast is still hot," I told him. "Someone said they might even be having scrambled eggs this morning."

"Mmm, that sounds good," he answered in an eager voice.

There are a few things about that whole scenario I find worth mentioning: Randy doesn't have an alarm clock in his room, but he was sharing in my feelings when he said he had done the same thing the day before; all laundry is placed in a large hamper in the soiled linen room, but referring to it as *his* laundry basket made it more personal; scrambled eggs are on the breakfast menu every morning and probably always will be, but boy was Randy excited.

I never knew what type of dementia Randy lived with because I found it irrelevant. My approach with each resident is not driven by diagnosis—it is driven by objective observation in the moment. There's an old saying that hits deep in the nursing field: "We treat the individual, not the disease."

I used that same tactical approach with Randy on several occasions, but due to his short-term memory loss, each time was brand new. As his dementia advanced over the months, I would need to adapt my approach to better fit his loss of capabilities and communication skills. Eventually, it got to the point where I was just telling him the story while washing and dressing him in his bed. I could tell by his cooperative movements and his attempts at joining in the story that his trust in me was still there.

There are other approaches I would use to get residents out of bed and ready for the day. I would ask Betty every morning if she would like coffee with her breakfast, and every morning she would answer with a resounding, "Yes, please." I didn't directly inform her that it was time to get up—the mention of coffee and breakfast was enough to convey the message. Even on mornings when she seemed less motivated, her "yes, please" would find its way out of her mouth, as though it had become a habit. Even under the attack of dementia, her brain was able to develop a new procedural practice. The same holds true for most of my morning routines with other residents. In her book *Thoughtful Dementia Care: Understanding the Dementia Experience*, Jennifer Ghent-Fuller describes this phenomenon in her chapter on procedural memory.

Here's another example: every morning I would ask Eric if he had socks on yet—adding the word "yet" was an implication that his socks were coming. Even though I knew he had no socks on, this was my prelude to pulling the lower edge of his blankets over his feet to have a look. Eric would instinctively throw the rest of the blankets off and pick up his feet. Other little procedures would follow in sequence: him sitting up on the side of his bed; him taking his top off and throwing it aside; me handing him a washcloth so he could wash his face; me putting a fresh shirt over his head; etc.

Eric didn't have the cognitive capacity to initiate this whole process, but he could easily cooperate in completing it. Without actually saying anything, I would encourage independence throughout the process. I would only jump in if he seemed to be having trouble with something. Putting on his shirt is a good example.

I noticed one morning that Eric was spending a bit more time getting his shirt on. I had put his shirt over his head, as usual, and he put one arm in his sleeve. As I was slipping his pants over his feet, Eric paused for a few seconds then took his first arm out of the sleeve. I'm guessing that in that moment of just a few seconds, his shirt went from being halfway on to being halfway off—he was simply trying to finish what he thought he had started.

"Did I put your shirt on backwards again?" I asked. I spun the shirt around his neck one full circle—in his mind, though, I had only spun it around halfway to correct my mistake. I didn't try to explain that he was in the middle of putting his shirt on; I didn't instruct him on how to put the other sleeve on; I didn't take over and put his shirt on for him—I simply admitted to a mistake that I never really made and carried on.

NUTRITION

The next task for the morning is getting the residents fed. Trying to explain to someone the importance of eating and drinking is like trying to tell them the importance of wearing a sweater on cold days—it's a bit patronizing. Also, every resident is given a clothing protector (essentially a bib) to prevent staining their clothes.

Not wanting them to feel like a toddler, I'll distract from the real reason for the clothing protector. "This should help keep your neck nice and warm," I tell them, as I fasten the snap.

Let's talk about Linda, the lady who was still full from the breakfast she never ate.

Linda never really resisted the LNAs when it came to getting washed and dressed—she was very cooperative and would carry on a conversation through the whole process. When it came to mealtime, however, Linda was one of the toughest nuts to crack.

Linda never liked to sit for too long—unless she was alone in her room and in her recliner. So, bringing her into a crowded dining room to sit on a semi-comfortable, non-reclining chair was often a challenge. I would often go to her room and tell her that her tablemates were wondering where she was. Other times I would tell her she had won a free breakfast, or whatever meal was being served. I might walk into her room with a shiver in my voice. "Well, they finally got the heater working in the dining room," I'd say to her as I pulled out a sweater from her closet. "Still, you should probably wear a sweater in there until it kicks in." Any of these approaches would usually at least get her to the dining room. Then came the issue of getting her to sit and stay seated until her meal was delivered.

I would usually walk with her to her table and pull up another chair for myself. "What am I thinking?" I'd say, with a slap to my forehead. "I forgot our breakfast—I'll be right back." I feel that calling it *our* breakfast compelled her to stay until I returned. I would return with her breakfast, telling her I could only carry one at a time, and tell her to start without me. I would walk away from the table and watch from a distance. Once she took her first bite, her mind was redirected toward her food; whether I returned or not was not an issue.

There were some residents who needed cueing or coaxing when it came to eating.

Donald would sometimes just sit and stare at his plate. Due to his cognitive decline, his brain wouldn't always make the connection between picking up his fork and using it to eat, even though he was quite capable of feeding himself. Rather than treat him like a toddler and ask him to pick up his fork, I would take a washcloth and wipe his hand. "What is all over your hand, Don?" I'd ask him. After wiping his hand—even though there was nothing on it—I would hand him his fork. "Here's your fork back," I'd tell him, suggesting that I had taken it away to wipe his hand.

Susan was often uninterested in eating—even her favorite meal could not entice her. We would try to inspire her by saying things like, "Oooh, lasagna, your favorite…" or "You must be starving, Sue…" One day, in an effort to at least get her started, I used her fork to pick up a small bite of turkey from her plate. In a cautious motion and in a wincey voice, I put it to her mouth. "Let's make sure this isn't too hot, Sue," I said to her, knowing very well it wasn't. "We wouldn't want to burn your tongue." She took her first bite.

"That's not too hot at all," she answered. I handed her the fork, and she took her second bite, then her third, and so on, until her plate was empty. The initial offering of the *"hot"* food got her mind focused on the temperature of the food, as opposed to the actual task of eating it. Once she got a taste, her mind was moved to how much she enjoyed it.

One resident, who lived most of her life in Philadelphia, could easily be inspired to eat by introducing each meal as "Philly" style: "Wow! Philly style pancakes..." or "Check out this Philly style meatloaf..." She seemed to enjoy every bite of every meal when it was Philly style.

Another reason some residents turn down a meal is because they think they have to pay for it. There are several tactical ways to distract them from the idea of having to pay. "I was told you paid ahead of time—smart move." Or, "This one's on the house; all you can eat." Those little follow-up anecdotes will usually distract them from the issue of having to pay—the first part of the phrase is trumped by the second part.

If a resident is known for continually worrying about paying for their meal, I will use tactical language and gestures to divert the issue of cost. I'll deliver a tablemate's meal first, telling them it's free breakfast Monday (or whatever day it might be). Then, I'll tell the concerned resident that I'll be right back with *their* free meal. Another tactic might be to write "paid" on their meal ticket and deliver it with their meal. There are many ways to deter from the issue of price; we just need to discover which tactics work with which residents.

Residents in the more advanced stages of their dementia require total assistance at mealtime. Often times they simply won't open their mouth. Dementia can have a taxing effect on the senses—food just doesn't smell or taste as good as it once did. In many cases, though, I find that sweets will arouse even the most stubborn tastebuds. Adding a bit of chocolate pudding to the tip of a spoonful of mashed potatoes and putting it to their lips will open almost any mouth. Some may think it's devious, teasing them with something sweet only to deliver something bland, but that little bit of sweetness is helping them stay nourished. Devious, perhaps. Tactical, yes. Compassionate, definitely.

Keeping the residents hydrated can also be a challenge; for some reason, they just do not pick up their cup. In this case, I might pour myself a small drink and propose a toast of some sort. "Let's have a toast to…" Or I might tell them I brought them the wrong drink. I'll bring them the "correct" drink and hand it to them while I remove the other drink from the table. The step between looking at the drink and actually picking it up has been skipped—the drink is off the table and in their hand. Often times, the drink I hand them is the same type of drink I remove from the table, but due to their dementia and calling it the "correct" drink, it becomes exactly that.

For those residents who require some assistance with their drinks, I prefer a narrow cup. I'll use a disposable cup and squeeze it a bit as I put it to their mouth. I feel the narrower tip of the cup causes an instinct to pucker their lips around it, and the drink doesn't end up spilling out the sides of their mouth like it does when they have to open their mouth wide.

Residents who require assistance and use a straw will sometimes let the straw just sit in their mouth—they don't automatically start drinking. In these cases, I will take an extra straw, dip it into their drink, and squeeze. With just a few drops of their drink in the straw, I will put it between their lips and let it go. That tiny bit of wetness in their mouth—and I do mean tiny—seems to stimulate them to keep drinking. I will immediately replace that straw with the one in their cup and they will keep right on drinking.

BATHING

One area of resident care where a tactical approach has proven to be helpful is bathing. Using a direct approach by telling a dementia resident they need a shower or bath—or even offering—can create unnecessary friction. They might feel insulted by you suggesting they are unclean; they might feel uncomfortable or embarrassed by the thought of being naked in front of a stranger; or they might feel incompetent, helpless, or insufficient.

As I mentioned earlier, I avoid any asking and offering. Instead, I will suggest the idea of a bath indirectly. "There's one person ahead of you for the bath, Sherry…I'll go see how much longer it's going to be." With the subject of the bath in the air, I'll walk out of the room, wait a minute or two, and then walk back in. "Wow! That was quick," I'll continue, making indirect references throughout the whole bathing and dressing process. "Let's be careful we don't get soap in your eyes…" as opposed to just telling her we need to wash her hair. "Where do you keep getting all these new clothes?" I'll ask, as I hand her one piece of clothing at a time.

I used to ask Paul, a landscaper by trade, whether he would rather have a warm bath or a cool bath; his dementia limited him to choosing between only what he was offered. Once he made his choice of a warm bath—of course—the actual bath itself was confirmed in his mind. I'd hold up two shirts and ask him which one he'd rather wear; I did the same with his pants. By having Paul be the one making those choices, he was confirming to himself that it was time to have a bath and get dressed. He also felt he was in control of the whole process.

One resident on the unit, Marie, always enjoyed a nice, warm bath. When it came time to wash her hair, though, her calm, relaxed demeanor was nowhere to be seen. On one occasion, halfway through her bath, I told Marie we wouldn't be able to wash her hair because I couldn't find her shampoo. "I could have sworn we put it back on the shelf last time," I said to her in confusion. This was to inspire a feeling that she was missing out on something.

Just before finishing her bath, I looked down toward the floor. "Oh, my goodness, Marie, look what I found." I picked up her bottle of shampoo—which was right where had I put it—and popped the top open.

"Wow," she replied, "nice work." I immediately wet her hair and began washing, keeping her mind occupied with little references to other subjects: how nice the shampoo smelled, how beautiful the weather was, etc. Her usual violent, aggravated, "don't touch my hair" attitude was kept at bay. Using this tactical approach with Marie, as devious as it may seem, not only allowed me to get her hair washed, but it also kept her from swinging into panic mode.

TOILETING

As beneficial as a tactical approach has proven to be when caring for people with dementia, one area of care where I consider it absolutely necessary is toileting.

A direct approach might include asking someone if they need to use the bathroom, which is something you might ask a three-year-old. For that reason alone, you're likely to get no for an answer.

Another direct approach might include telling them directly that they had an "accident"—this will likely cause them to feel ashamed and embarrassed. As good as your intentions may be, it's hard to be direct and discreet at the same time.

I'd like to share some of the tactical approaches I use when toileting residents with dementia. Before we begin, though, understand that I had built and maintained a friendly relationship with each of these residents.

OUTSIDE THE BOX

Peggy, despite her dementia, still had good control of her bowel and bladder, toileting herself throughout the day. She wore regular underwear with no pad or liner. As competent as she was at getting to the toilet on time, though, she wasn't as competent when it came to wiping herself. I was sure she would resist if I told her directly that I needed to check if her bottom was clean.

One morning, while Peggy was in the bathroom, I stood outside with a few wipes in my hand. "Peggy," I said when she came out, "just the person I was looking for." I told her it was Thursday, again, and that the nurse had asked me to do her weekly check of her feet and her bottom. She sighed a bit but didn't argue. We walked back into the bathroom where she pulled down her britches and sat back on the toilet. I pulled off her slippers and gave her feet a quick once-over with one of the wipes. "Your feet look good," I told her. "Let's hope your bottom does too." She stood up and patiently waited while I wiped her bottom. I kept the dirty wipes out of her sight; there was no need for her to feel embarrassed. "No problems there, either. You're taking really good care of yourself. Nice work."

The fact that it was Thursday had nothing to do with anything, but it created a reason why I was there. The nurse didn't actually ask me to check on Peggy, but it sounded more official. Her feet did not really need to be checked, but including and checking her feet first led her to accept the idea that her bottom was next. By using a wipe on her feet, she was not surprised when I used them on her bottom. Complimenting how well she was taking care of herself was just a little positive reinforcement, something we all need.

Next, there's Michael. Michael would take himself to the bathroom and was continent most of the time. In light of those occasional episodes of incontinence, though, the nurses and Mike's family thought it would be best if he wore Pull-Ups—to him they were just warm underwear.

Someone once put a sticky-tab brief (a diaper) on Michael after finding he had wet himself, but that quickly proved to be impractical. One morning, just after breakfast, he brought himself to the bathroom and pulled his pants and brief down as usual. When he tried pulling everything back up, the brief just wouldn't stay—pulling it down past his hips had caused the sticky tabs to loosen up. So, he did what anyone with a diminished level of judgement would do: he took it off, threw it on the floor, and pulled his pants up.

Asking him directly to come to the bathroom to put on a fresh pair of underwear was usually met with, "I'm all set, thanks." A tactical approach was always more effective.

A few times each day, I would grab a Pull-Up from Mike's drawer and track him down. "Hey, Mike, I finally found you the right size underwear," I'd tell him. "They're the same exact size that I wear…what a coincidence."

We'd go into the bathroom, and he'd have a seat on the toilet with his pants and "underwear" down.

If his Pull-Up was wet, I would pretend to look at the back label to check the size. "Yup, one size too big. These should fit you much better," referring to the new Pull-Up, which was actually the same size. I'd swap out the Pull-Ups, help him wash up, and send him on his way.

On the other hand, if his Pull-Up was still clean, I would face the other way and kill a few minutes by looking at my assignment sheet and making a few marks with my pen while he sat on the toilet. These marks were just scribbles, but my looking busy allowed him not to feel like he was being watched. Most times the mere act of sitting on the toilet would trigger his bowel or bladder or both. I would help him wash up and send him on his way. The fresh Pull-Up—or right-size underwear—never came into play; I simply returned it to his drawer.

Sam, a house painter back in the day, was another resident whose incontinence came and went at different times on different days. I could usually get him to head towards the bathroom by asking his opinion on what color we should paint the walls. Asking his opinion made him feel valued. On the way to the bathroom, though, I would divert the conversation into something else to do with the bathroom. Getting a clean brief out his drawer, I'd lead him into the bathroom and tell him the seat might be a little cold. Wiping the seat to warm it up for him was all the subliminal hinting needed to get him to sit. From that point on, his mind was on the real reason for us being there. The challenge with Sam wasn't toileting; it was getting him to the bathroom to begin with.

Many residents on the dementia unit are quite capable of finding the bathroom, but they no longer possess the mental capacity to follow the many steps involved with toileting oneself. Many are in wheelchairs and simply can't transfer to the toilet without assistance, whether it be physically or mechanically—this is where incontinence runs rampant.

When one of these residents has an episode of incontinence, the last thing they need is a direct approach—they don't need to be told they had an "accident" and need to be changed. What they need is to be taken care of without being made to feel degraded. They need an indirect, distracting, and tactical approach that will coax them into the bathroom while allowing them to maintain their dignity.

Barbara, who needed minor assistance in the bathroom, was on a medication that would cause her to have loose stools now and then. These episodes would occur at random times of the day, and we were unable to establish a routine toileting time to beat her to the punch, so to say. I'd bring her to the bathroom and position her in front the toilet—she had a tendency to sit before she was lined up properly with the toilet. "Uh-oh!" I'd say as I brought her pants down, "It looks like you might be getting that bug that's been going around. I know how you feel—I had the same thing yesterday." With her dignity still intact, she was relieved that she wasn't the only one. "You'll probably feel much better tomorrow," I told her.

Hands-on assistance might be refused for the simple reason that it's just that—hands on. The resident might not want to be touched. An elusive reference to the bathroom on the way there can minimize any anxiety they might experience once they get there. "I hope they unclogged your toilet by now…I had the same problem yesterday." Or, "We should probably get to the bathroom before someone else beats us there…that seems to be the busiest room in the house." Or, "I'll look for those pants you wanted while you're in the bathroom…I'm guessing they put them in your bottom drawer." As I stated earlier, those little follow-up anecdotes can act as a buffer—they soften the blow of the initial reference to the bathroom without changing the subject.

Refusing mechanical assistance by use of a sit-to-stand machine rarely has anything to do with the toilet, but with how intimidating the machine appears to some residents. Rather than explain to them that the machine is harmless and that they must wear the harness in order for the machine to help them stand, I put the focus on whether or not the harness will fit them. "We'd better make sure this belt fits you before we hook it to the lift," I'd tell them, even though it's pretty much one-size-fits-all. "Can you lean forward just a tad?" I'd ask. Once the harness is on, I'll ask the resident if it's too tight.

"That actually fits pretty good," or something along that line is a common response. If they say it's too tight—even though I know it's not—I'll pretend to readjust it and ask if it feels better. "Much better." Their focus is no longer on the intimidating machine in front of them, but on the comfort of the harness. The actual task of toileting becomes secondary.

Even residents who are totally dependent and can only be changed in bed can be resistant. The first time I helped one of the other aides change Bruce in his bed, he was very resistant to being rolled to either side. He had no idea we were there to get him washed and into some clean clothes, and he may have felt he was being manhandled for no particular reason.

The next time we put Bruce in his bed to be changed, I decided to use a tactical approach. "Hey, Bruce, are you right-handed or left-handed?" I asked him.

"Right-handed," he answered.

"Well then, let's roll to your right first," I said to him. If Bruce had told me he was left-handed, I would still have suggested rolling to his right first; his answer was irrelevant. Also, using the word "first" conveyed a silent message that we would be rolling to his left next.

MEDICATION

Every resident on the unit is on some type of medication. While most are agreeable when the nurse brings their medication, some can be resistant at times.

Dennis, who I mentioned earlier, saw no need to take his scheduled pain medicine for pain he wasn't feeling; his dementia kept him from foreseeing the inevitable pain in his near future. This pain would usually manifest itself in mood swings. The longer he resisted, the more elevated his anxiety became. Every attempt at explaining the benefits of taking his pain pills led to even higher levels of anxiety.

Knowing I had developed a close, friendly relationship with Dennis during his stay, one of the nurses asked me to intervene. According to New Hampshire Revised Statute Section (NH RSA) 326-B:14, an LNA is authorized to administer medication if a licensed nurse supervises the procedure. After waiting several minutes and allowing him to settle down, I sat at his table and took an obvious look at my watch. I told Dennis it was almost time for his pain meds. "...I just need to be sure they're not out of date..." While the nurse supervised from a distance, I handed Dennis his meds and told him the juice to wash it down might be a bit cold.

Telling him it was *almost* time for his pain meds put a subtle hint in the air. Telling him I needed to be sure the pills weren't out of date was another indirect reference to the idea of pills. Also, the idea that the juice might be a bit cold had him paying attention to the juice even more than the pills.

Another resident who proved to be a struggle when the nurses were passing medications was Marge. After an assessment of Marge's ability to swallow large pills, it was decided that her pills would be crushed and mixed with something sweet—Marge really loved her sweets. While crushing the pills would certainly make them easier to swallow, the pill crusher had its limits and there were always chunks in the sweet mixture. Often times Marge would simply suck the sauce out of the mixture then spit out the leftover unwanted chunks of medicine.

Knowing this was an ongoing challenge with Marge, I carried a wrapper from a crunchy candy bar in my pocket. "Wow!" I said, as I showed her the wrapper and put the spoon to her mouth. "I love these crunchy candy bars... Enjoy!" The sight of that very familiar wrapper made that spoonful of chunky chocolate a bit more appetizing.

"Mmm, that *is* good," she said, as she took in that spoonful of sweetened medicine, chunks and all. The fact that I wasn't actually holding a candy bar but a spoonful of chocolate syrup was irrelevant—her mind was occupied with the taste.

Many residents on the unit are on some type of pain medication, which can cause constipation. Although it's not considered a medication, per se, prune juice is considered a necessary, unappetizing commodity. Unfortunately, the bitter taste will turn most folks off after the very first sip, and explaining the reason for the prune juice is not likely to change a resident's taste buds.

I always stir a bit of sweetener into the juice beforehand and offer the resident some of our new "blueberry" juice. This suggestive persuasion is usually enough to get them to take that first sip.

If I feel a bit of trickery might be needed, I might hold the drink behind my back and ask them to "...pick a hand, any hand..." then present them their prize. Or I might ask them to pick a number from one to three. Believe it or not, they get it right every time; go figure. Alternatively, I might bring a drink of my own and join them in a toast. Whatever approach I use, I avoid telling them directly why they need the prune juice in the first place.

BEHAVIORS

Up to now, we've concentrated on the physical aspects of caring for residents with dementia and what they might refuse. We've discussed some of the benefits a tactical approach can bring as opposed to a direct, matter-of-fact approach. We've gone over the importance of building a relationship with residents because it inspires trust and encourages cooperation. Now let's talk about what is likely the deciding factor for many families when considering a nursing home for their loved one with dementia.

When it comes to washing, dressing, feeding, and toileting their loved one at home—as stressful as it might be—most families do an amazing job. It is most often the behavioral aspect of the dementia that causes families to reach out beyond family and friends for assistance.

Gary's wife was overwhelmed by his constant wandering to the basement to see what was making that hissing sound—she could not convince him that it was the furnace cycling on and off. She felt compelled to look into a nursing home when he began to be suspicious of noises coming from outside that were mostly from traffic on their busy road.

Brenda's daughters both had jobs and families, so they did not have the time to watch over their mother's dangerous compulsion to always be "cooking something up for everyone." As scary as her behavior was during the daytime, the real concern for Brenda's safety came during the overnight hours. Knowing that nursing homes work on a twenty-four-hour basis, the daughters decided a nursing home was the best option for the entire family.

David was brought to the nursing home when he started to continually ask his wife who she was and why she was in his house. With his long-term memory being the driving factor in his life, David was living his life as if it were thirty years earlier—he no longer recognized the eighty-year-old woman standing in his kitchen as his wife.

Although it's difficult to label behaviors under the same category as something residents might refuse, a tactical approach—as opposed to being direct and straightforward—can still be applied when dealing with adverse behaviors. We use distraction, redirection, pacification, and a whole slew of other devices to gain their attention, ease any anxiety, and foster a more positive, more agreeable environment. Let's discuss a few of these behaviors a bit deeper.

EXIT SEEKING

As the old saying goes, There's no place like home. It's no wonder many residents on the dementia unit often go through what we call exit seeking. They'll stand at the locked exit door and repeatedly push, push, push in an effort to get out. They'll punch in combination after combination trying to unlock it. Allowing their unresolved effort to continue too long can lead to elevated levels of anxiety, frustration, and anger.

Approaching an exit seeking resident in a direct manner, patiently and calmly explaining that the doors are locked to keep them safe, will likely stir feelings of inferiority and humility. It may convey a message that they cannot fend for themselves. The use of a tactical approach—redirecting their attention without ignoring their feelings—will prove more effective.

"Is that door still broken?" I'll ask the resident while pushing on the door. "I put in a work request for this door yesterday...looks like we might need to put another one in, huh?" Me pushing on the door not only puts us on the same page, but it also shows that their situation is not being ignored.

Another approach I use is to suggest that we try the door at the other end of the hallway. On the way, I'll introduce other points that have absolutely nothing to do with getting out. "Will you be watching the big game tonight?" Or, "Any idea what we're having for lunch today?" Putting these points in the form of a question causes their mind to consider an answer, distracting them from the whole idea of the "broken" door.

All residents considered to be an exit risk are fitted with a wander-guard, a small device that sets off an alarm when it's within range of an opened exit door. Some are placed on the wrist, others on the ankle, and others on the resident's walker. Regardless of their placement, wander-guards are often an unwelcome amenity. Residents will go to great lengths to get them off. One supervisor of mine allowed me to carry an out-of-order wander-guard with me. It was fitted with a rubber band, allowing me to put it on and remove it at will. Before any argument would ensue about wanting theirs removed, I would slip mine on and point out that I had the same bracelet or anklet as them, following up with something like, "Where'd you get yours...?"

One resident, Hazel, did manage to make it through the exit door once. She followed a member of the cleaning crew through the door as they were exiting the unit.

The alarm *did* sound, but there was no one in the area to guide her back. I caught up with her on the next unit over. "Hazel," I called out to her, "I found those pants you've been looking for. Guess where they were?" This little white lie motivated her to come with me to her room, where I pulled out a random pair of pants and showed them to her. She was so happy to have her pants back, which were never really missing.

Not all exit seeking involves an actual attempt to leave the building. One resident, Walter, would often tell me he had to get home to get the house cleaned up. Learning that Walter had a sister through our conversations during morning care, I informed him that Phyllis had already taken care of it. "I think she even did a load of your laundry." Phyllis was well aware of this tactic and was very appreciative. She knew her brother would not stand for someone telling him he couldn't go home, no matter how delicate their words might be.

Tina, another verbal exit seeker, had lived in the same apartment building for the past several years. Much like those residents who worried about paying for their lunch, she would often worry about paying her rent. "Your rent is all paid up for the next two weeks," I'd tell her. "That means you'll probably be getting your next bill within a few days."

Telling her that she would be getting her *next* bill was a subliminal message that her previous bill was all set. Adding the words "within a few days" assured her she would be here when it arrived—or at least for a few more days. I wasn't worried about her approaching me the next day and asking me about her bill. Knowing how affected her short-term memory had become, the very mention of receiving her next bill would be forgotten within the next few minutes.

Tom would exit seek both physically and verbally, as he was sure he didn't belong in the facility. I asked the social worker to print up a mailing label for him, changing the words "Nursing Home" to "Place." I feel the words "Nursing Home" carry an end-of-life message, so changing this would help Tom feel more at ease. The label looked very official:

Tom Smith
Sunrise Place
Somewhere, NH 55555

I put that label on a car magazine from the facility lobby and brought it to Tom's room, telling him he had mail. That magazine, with that official-looking label, raised Tom's self-awareness—he was somebody. It also gave him a connection to the outside world while subliminally reinforcing the idea that this was his mailing address, that this was where he lived. I topped it off by telling him I loved what he'd done with the place. Tom was not exit seeking when I brought him his mail, but why wait?

WANDERING AND RUMMAGING

It's not unusual on any given day to see a number of residents pacing the halls of the unit. Some might be on their way to their room, while others are simply not interested in whatever entertainment might be going on. Some may be on their way to the bathroom—which is always a safe assumption—but need guidance and assistance. Some, however, are on an endless, trivial mission with no real destination. They enter other residents' rooms; they sit in their chairs; they lie on their beds; and they go through their things. In short, they wander and rummage.

Let's take another look at Phil, the man who was sifting through his roommate's closet. As I mentioned earlier, we had recently caught Phil several times on Joe's side of the room. He wasn't being nosey, and he wasn't trying to steal anything. He was repeating a process he had gotten used to when he was in his previous room. If Phil had been in some other room, sifting through someone else's things, I would consider him to be wandering and rummaging.

Andrea, on the other hand, was a wanderer. She was not considered a fall risk. So, aside from leading her into her bathroom a few times a day for toileting, we pretty much let her be, as it was good exercise for her. Andrea had a habit of entering other residents' rooms and adding something to the basket on her walker—she seemed to prefer small stuffed animals.

One resident who *was* aware of Andrea's comings and goings was Louise. She would walk right up to Andrea and try to explain that the items in her basket didn't belong to her. As peaceful and respectful as Louise spoke, though, Andrea refused to give up what she thought was hers. A small back-and-forth argument would ensue and could very easily become hostile. To have a staff member jump in and tell Andrea the same thing Louise had just told her would simply create a two against one predicament, and Andrea might become even more defensive. Trying to explain Andrea's wandering to Louise might be mistaken as us excusing Andrea's behavior. Each of those direct approaches ends with someone feeling snubbed, and we end up being the bad guy.

I chose to redirect Louise's attention away from those objects that didn't belong to Andrea. I grabbed one of Louise's many stuffed animals from her room and jumped into the still nonviolent argument, grabbing one of the stuffed animals from Andrea's basket. I held up the two items to show Louise. "Is one of these yours?" I asked. She quickly picked out the one I had pulled from her room. I showed the label to Andrea, pointing out Louise's name. I told her it looked just like the one she had. "My wife has one just like it," I added.

Once Louise pointed out her own stuffed animal, thinking we had recovered it, the rest of the items in the basket were of little concern; she went to her room and put it back on her bureau. I didn't bother returning the other stuffed animals to their rightful owners; instead, I asked Andrea if she would help me deliver some animals from lost and found to their homes. She was more than happy to help.

AGGRESSION

When a resident with dementia becomes aggressive, we don't automatically assume they're angry. They might be in pain and don't know how to communicate and ask for help; they may be having a reaction to a certain medication; they may have a urinary tract infection or some other condition that causes mood swings; they may be reexperiencing an unpleasant incident from their past; or it could be something as trivial as being hungry. Uncovering the cause of the aggression and allowing the nurse to treat it can prove difficult. Whatever the cause may be, aggression can cause residents to become even more resistant to accepting care.

A direct, straightforward approach might involve trying to calm the resident down through talking; however, the resident may not feel they are being aggressive and therefore disregard anything you say. The resident might even become more aggressive because they might feel they're being patronized.

I remember one resident, Charlie, trying to carry on a conversation with another resident, Lucy, whose dementia had taken away the better part of her communication skills. Although she could still pronounce words clearly, she was unable to put meaningful words in a meaningful order to form a meaningful sentence.

Charlie sat in the chair beside Lucy and asked her something about her wheelchair—I believe it had something to do with the footrests. Lucy's answer was a jumble of random words: "Munching valley from seven on licorice." Those weren't her actual words, but you get the picture. He asked her the same question again and got another jumbled answer. His next question wasn't as pleasant, and a bit louder.

"What the hell are you talking about?" he yelled. He got yet another jumbled, monotone answer. All that mumbling and jumbling was clearly causing a bit of frustration for Charlie—you could see it in his eyes. His dementia kept him from grasping the idea that Lucy was incapable of giving a straight answer, so he kept right on asking questions, expecting an answer that made sense. I had to step in before Charlie's frustration morphed into aggression.

I didn't ask Charlie to leave Lucy alone, and I didn't try to explain Lucy's condition to him. I pulled up another chair and started moving Lucy's footrests in all kinds of ways, acting as though I was performing an inspection. "Oh, my goodness, Charlie," I said to him. "How did you even notice that?" I removed one of Lucy's footrests and showed it to him. "This thing needs to be tightened up—do you have a wrench that would fit this?" My tone of voice and body language gave off a sense of urgency.

"I'm not sure," he told me. Charlie's concern was no longer focused on Lucy's muddled answers. We walked toward his room and talked about different things, anything to get his mind off of Lucy. Being about his same size, I asked if I might be able to borrow one of his shirts for a job interview. Not only did he say it would be okay, but he even helped me pick it out. I had no intention of borrowing his shirt, but the boost in his self-esteem was very noticeable—he had something I needed and was happy to oblige.

I coaxed him into using the bathroom one last time before we headed back to the TV room. Helping him get his pants down, I "accidently" tore one of the sticky-tabs on his brief, which was a little wet. I grabbed a fresh brief from his closet and helped him get it on. In his mind I wasn't replacing his brief because it was wet—which he was unaware of—but I was replacing it because I "accidently" ripped it. We returned to the TV room, walking right past Lucy, and joined the rest of the folks to watch a movie.

REPETITIVENESS

Several times throughout the day, many residents on the dementia unit will go through a cycle of repetitiveness. Whether it be organizing things in their room, making their bed, repeated questions, or any number of other things, their dementia has them doing and saying things repeatedly. When they do or say anything meaningful to them—which could literally be anything—their short-term memory loss prevents them from remembering that they've already done it or said it.

On the subject of short-term memory, I might sometimes forget if I already did something of significance. For instance, I might forget if I switched my laundry from the washer to the dryer. To be on the safe side, I'll go to the laundry room to check—most times my clothes were still in the washer. Having verified the clothing situation, my short-term memory can rest easy. This does not hold true for dementia residents.

OUTSIDE THE BOX

When a resident is continuously reorganizing things in their room, for instance, they don't quite remember where they started and it becomes a perpetual cycle. If that resident is safely being active, I don't deter them—being active is a good thing. If, however, there seems to be any risk involved in their reorganizing efforts or if that resident is supposed to be somewhere else, I will join in to finish their task, compliment their work, and coax them into joining me for lunch, a snack, or anything else that will draw them away from the scene.

Asking them to stop or trying to explain that everything is where it belongs might confuse them even more—how would *I* know where *their* things go? It could also provoke a "mind your own business" response.

One resident, Amy, would make and remake her bed several times a day. Aside from her scheduled physical therapy sessions, this was the only exercise she got that involved different muscle groups. She wasn't deemed a fall risk, so there was no immediate danger. I watched from the hallway one day as she was remaking her bed. From the pictures on the wall, I could see she had served in the military. Having been there before, I knew how meticulous drill sergeants were when it came to bedmaking—they were hard to please. When she had finished making her bed, I would walk into her room and look it over. "Nice work," I'd tell her. "Now, let's go have some lunch." She was never really able to make her bed up to military standards, so I would usually go back to her room while she was eating and do some touch-up to her bed.

If repetitiveness were an Olympic event, the gold medal would have to go to asking the same question time, after time, after time, and so on. People with dementia live in a world of confusion and uncertainty; they look for answers wherever they might find them, and a few minutes later they're looking for those answers again. Telling them they've already asked a certain question is of little help—not only did they forget asking the question, but they also forgot that you already answered it.

One lady, Dorothy, would continuously ask, "Kevin, what am I doing wrong?" Instead of simply telling her she was doing nothing wrong, which would lead to the question being repeated, I would come up with something minor and help her resolve the issue. If she was wearing a button up shirt, for example, I would stand directly in front of her and give her a quick once over. My body language would prompt her to stand still—she didn't want to interfere with my inspection.

"Aha," I'd say to her, "somebody missed a button on your shirt." I'd reach over, undo a couple of buttons, and do them back up. As far as she was concerned, whatever was wrong was now fixed.

I often wondered how Dorothy's short-term memory—or lack thereof—could cause her to forget asking a question while allowing her to remember my name. Looking back, I believe it had much to do with our relationship and what I like to call emotional instinct. I feel that her trust in me caused something, somewhere in her head to hold onto my name.

To demonstrate the power of this so-called emotional instinct, I'll share a short story that had Dorothy's daughter both traumatized and elated at the same time.

One afternoon, while her daughter was visiting, I entered Dorothy's room to restock a few items. I didn't want to disturb their time together, so I just gave a quick "hello." Suddenly, Dorothy's daughter came right out and asked her, "Mom, what's my name?" She was attempting to jar her mother's memory. After a brief moment of silence, Dorothy turned and looked over to me.

"Kevin, what's her name?" she asked. As traumatized as she was, Dorothy's daughter was impressed with her mom's ability to remember someone's name, even if it wasn't hers.

THE LIST GOES ON

Exit seeking, wandering, aggression, and repetitiveness are just a few examples from the inexhaustible list of behaviors you might find in people with dementia; however, looking at these few examples should be enough to show that a tactical approach, as opposed to being direct and up-front, can work wonders. We can't instruct people how to behave, and we can't reason with people whose cognitive capacities have been compromised by dementia. We can, however, distract and redirect their attention to focus on something totally off the subject that may be causing their behavior.

BUILDING AND MAINTAINING RELATIONSHIPS

I can only imagine the lonely, confusing, frightening world that dementia residents live in. They wile away the hours unaware of what day it is, trying to make sense of their surroundings and looking for someone or something familiar to help them feel secure. We can help ease their anxiety and loneliness by building and maintaining a friendly relationship with each of them. Unlike the complexities involved in building a relationship with our peers—which requires active participation from both parties—building a relationship with these residents can be accomplished almost instantly, much like the way I did with Jack, the graduate of Dover High School who I never really shared a class with.

In my eighteen years of working with folks living with dementia, I have never met a family member or friend who was unwilling to share little bits of information that would help me break the ice between the resident and myself—where they grew up, what kind of work they did, etc. Other useful information about a person can be gathered through simple observation of items in their room: they're a sports fan; they have children; they have pictures of places they've traveled to. All these seemingly tiny bits of information can become the key to a door they've been wanting someone to open, they just didn't know how to give it away or who to give it to.

Maintaining these relationships is essential to gaining more and more of their trust. As their trust grows, so grows their cooperation during care—so grows their self-esteem and their quality of life.

In the midst of all my traveling throughout the unit each day, I like to acknowledge each resident I pass along the way—a simple nod of the head while I say their name is sufficient. If I have a few seconds, I'll stop and offer a compliment or an uplifting comment. "Where can I get a hat like that, Joe?" Or, "I see you've been to the hairdresser, Julie. Nice!"

I would tell Martha on a daily basis that my wife said hello, "Tell Martha I said hello..." I'd say, in my best impression of my wife's friendly voice.

"Awe," she'd reply with a smile. "She's such a nice girl."

"I'll tell her you said 'hi.'" Did my wife actually say hello? No. But that little five-second exchange gave Martha a friend somewhere outside the facility—a friend she had never even met.

Allen always seemed uplifted whenever I'd ask if I could borrow one of his shirts. "You gotta let me borrow that shirt sometime, Al—my wife would love it." I had no intention of borrowing any of Allen's shirts, but I was a friend in need; therefore, I was a friend indeed.

SUMMARY

When providing care for nursing home residents, we must consider the Nursing Home Reform Act of 1987, which states that nursing home residents have the right to refuse care of any kind, at any time, for any reason—this applies to all residents regardless of mental acuity.

When a resident's mental capacity is intact, any refusal of care will usually come with a reasonable explanation—perhaps they're not hungry at mealtime, or perhaps they'd rather wait a while before getting dressed for the day. We respect their right to refuse and reapproach a bit later.

On the other hand, when a resident living with dementia refuses care, it often comes with no reason at all—none that makes sense, anyway. Professionally, we are obligated to respect their right to refuse, while ethically, we are obligated to give our best effort to turn these refusals around.

Trying to explain, reason, inform, or instruct these residents into accepting care can lead to elevated levels of anxiety, embarrassment, and aggression. These emotions and reactions can be minimized if we build and maintain a relationship with each resident.

To dispute the wisdom of an old adage—with regards to treating dementia residents—honesty is not the best policy. Be tactical; be creative; think outside the box.

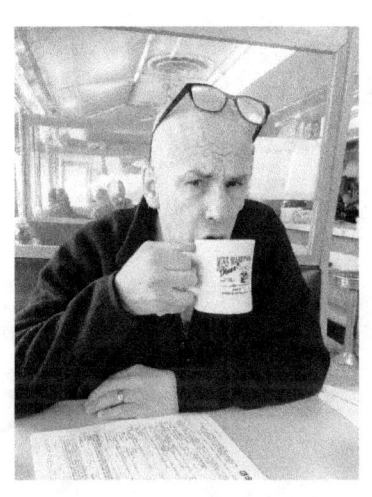
Kevin Walters, LNA, brings 18 years of experience in dementia care, both in nursing homes and in-home settings. His work is inspired by the personal care refusals he encountered from dementia residents. Walters is the author of T.O.M and several essays published in NHTI's "The Eye". Married to Kelly since 1996, he is a father of six and a grandfather of two. In 2021, he settled in Center Barnstead, NH. Outside of his professional life, Kevin is a member of St. Katherine Drexel Parish and enjoys cooking, writing, and Wednesday night poker. His latest book, Outside the Box, is a valuable resource for professional caregivers and families alike.

www.ingramcontent.com/pod-product-compliance
Lightning Source LLC
LaVergne TN
LVHW020527140126
829810LV00010B/791